Chair exercises for Seniors

Contents

INTRODUCTION

Exercising regularly is critical for all of us, no matter what age we are, but in particular for those who are already over 50. Regular exercise keeps our bodies moving and ensures that they continue to work effectively as we age, regardless of whether or not we love it. If we don't move around and keep our muscles active, our chances of growing older healthily are significantly diminished.

Your elderly friend or family member could enjoy working out, but they've probably always been told that it's good for them, regardless of how they feel about it. What if they are now encountering an impediment to their mobility? In their younger years, they may have been able to run 10 miles a day or compete in a triathlon; however, now, it is just becoming more difficult for them to stand.

Suppose an older adult is having difficulty getting around on their own and is finding it difficult to get even a little amount of exercise during the day. In that case, they shouldn't worry too much because there are still ways to exercise without budging from a chair!

Chair exercises are an excellent alternative for seniors. There is no requirement for a weight set, a personal trainer, or even constant supervision from a caregiver regarding seniors engaging in physical activity. The only thing a senior need is a chair; however, several of the following exercises may require a resistance band or dumbbells to be performed precisely and achieve the desired effects.

Please remember that everyone's comfort level varies greatly when exercising. You must start slowly and establish a fitness regimen specific to your capabilities to avoid injury.

The Advantages of Chair Exercise

Not only will a regular exercise routine (ideally consisting of at least 30 minutes per day) keep the heart healthy in an elderly adult, but it can help avoid other serious health problems, such as high blood pressure, strokes, heart attacks, falls, and chronic disorders like dementia.

Some of the benefits you are certain to enjoy from doing etiquette chair exercises include the following, which is not an exhaustive list.

Perfect Posture: Your muscles will be in the ideal position if you have perfect posture, which is achieved by sitting up perfectly straight on the chair. Your body would be revitalized, and you would no longer have feelings of fatigue as a result.

Pain Reduction: Most chair exercises have as their primary objective the reduction of pain and stiffness in the joints, as well as the relaxation of tense muscles.

Increased Flexibility: When the limbs are appropriately stretched, you will find that the muscles become more supple, which will result in increased flexibility. Your body will become more flexible, allowing you to maintain a physically active and fit lifestyle.

Improved Coordination: The repetitive nature of chair exercises helps achieve Coordination of muscle groups and ensures that your spine is aligned properly. This results in better Coordination. Because the processes are repeated, even older adults with dementia can remember them.

Improved Circulation: If you continue to perform chair exercises regularly, you should see an improvement in your lung capacity. This improves your mobility and helps wounds heal more quickly, shortening the time needed for recovery.

Improved Stability: Because you regularly exercise chair, your body has improved stability. Falling and injuring oneself physically will be less likely due to this.

Build self-confidence: Acquiring self-confidence means that you can handle several tasks at the same time without worrying about traveling from one location to another. The newly acquired sense of self-assurance contributes to the improvement of mental health.

Although those over 50+ may not be able to move quickly or even get out of their seats, this should not prevent them from engaging in physical activity. Many standard workouts can be performed while utilizing a chair as a mode of mobility.

Seniors can still attain all the advantages mentioned earlier using a standard chair. They don't need to purchase something new to begin moving around; all that is required is an ordinary chair. This chair should have four legs for stability, no wheels or rollers, and it should not have arms for most activities.

We have compiled a comprehensive list of activities that older adults can perform in the privacy and convenience of their own homes, utilizing only the apparatus they can operate independently. We will break down each exercise into its components and demonstrate how to carry out each using concrete examples.

We're not presenting a one-size-fits-all list. Injuries may make some workouts impossible or necessitate a complete cessation of participation. When a senior is experiencing pain, it should not be assumed that they can perform a specific exercise. If this happens, they must immediately return to their original position and terminate the practice.

Take caution if you're a caregiver for an older adult and are unsure whether or not you're allowed to perform any of the following activities. With the help of visual aids, the chair exercises for the seniors are explained in detail. It is imperative that you perform each exercise according to the prescribed number of reps, sets, and duration.

SECTION ONE

ARM EXERCISES

Shoulders

Shoulders serve a very wide variety of functions for humans. Our shoulders bear enormous loads; some of us sleep on them; we tumble and lean on them; throughout the day, we engage in various activities that need us to move our shoulders in several ways. Shoulder exercises have a significant positive impact on our overall capabilities when it comes to using our arms.

Suppose a senior cannot have a full range of motion in their shoulders or even a minimal amount of shoulder range of motion. In that case, they may experience a lack of strength, pain in other parts of their body for picking up the slack, or a reduced ability to function in their day-to-day activities. Even a minimal amount of shoulder range of motion can be detrimental.

Shoulder Press

Complicacy	Reps /Sets	Minimum Time
Easy	8-12/2-3	4 minutes

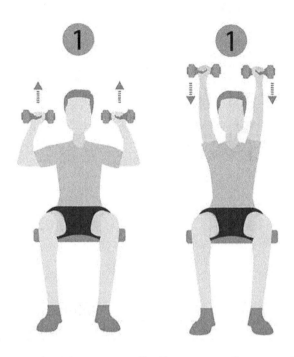

Strength, mobility, and endurance will all improve from performing seated shoulder presses. This will help stretch the arms upward.

Steps:

1. Choose a set of light dumbbells to exercise, slip a resistance band under the seat, or sit on the band while maintaining an even length on both sides of the body.

2. Place your hips as far back as they will go in the chair while maintaining a comfortable sitting position. Check that the chair's back is firmly attached to the backrest.

3. Maintain a tight core by contracting the abs and lumbar region.

4. To start, begin with both elbows splayed to the sides of the body and then line them underneath the shoulders. Put some space between your ribs.

5. Maintain a neutral spine, hands facing front, and a firm hold on the dumbbells.

6. Reach your arms up and above your head until they are completely extended in this position (or get to a range that feels most comfortable). It is important to avoid touching the palms of the hands together and keep the arms in a parallel position.

7. After reaching the maximum extent of the arm's extension, bring the hands back to the starting position as gently as possible while maintaining a wide elbow stance. Instead of bringing the elbows toward the middle of the body, you should extend them outward until the top of the back feels a pinching sensation (which should not be painful) near the shoulder blades.

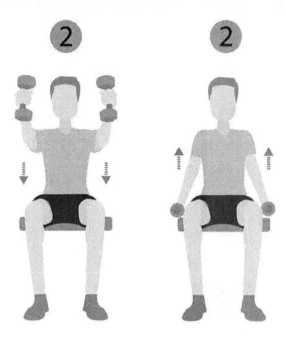

Front Shoulder Raises

Complicacy	Reps /Sets	Minimum Time
Easy	8-12/2-3	4 minutes

This exercise is very helpful for holding objects in front of the body or extending an arm forward, as it strengthens the muscles that support those movements.

Steps:

1. Grab some dumbbells, a resistance band, or a medicine ball, and get ready to work out.
2. Place your hips as far back as they will go in the chair while maintaining a comfortable sitting position. Check that the chair's back is firmly attached to the backrest.
3. Maintain a tight core by contracting the abs and lumbar region. Put some space between your ribs.
4. When doing out with dumbbells, maintain your arms by your sides and let them hang naturally, with both palms pointing inward toward the body.
5. You may adjust the length of a resistance band by sliding it under the seat or sitting on it until it is the same distance from your body on both sides. The next step is to retain both arms by your sides, allowing them to hang freely while keeping your palms facing inward toward your body.
6. When using a medicine ball, position the ball so it rests on the edge of the lap. With both hands, maintain a firm grasp on the ball while keeping the other hand on each side.
7. Continue to bring the arms up in front of the body while maintaining the arms' straight position and the palms' position, so they face inward.

8. When the arms are in a position where they are parallel to the floor, and the hands are in a position where they can be seen directly by the eyes, the motion should be stopped.
9. Proceed to return to the position you were in before slowly.

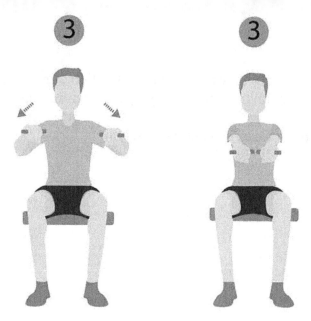

Chest

Seated Chest Press (Positioned)

Complicacy	Reps /Sets	Minimum Time
Easy	8-12/2-3	4 minutes

This type of exercise, which works not only the chest muscles but also the shoulders and the triceps, is referred to as a compound movement because it engages different muscle groups simultaneously.

Steps:

1. Get yourself a band of resistance.
2. Position the resistance band on the chair so that it is directly behind the back, right below the area that would be the shoulder blades. It is important to ensure that the resistance band does not have any room to move while it is attached to the back of the chair; if it moves at all, it could cause an injury or target the wrong muscle areas. Consider using a sturdy clip or pin to keep it in place, or have a member of the senior's family assist them in installing a pair of shelving brackets to the back of the chair so that the band remains in the appropriate position.
3. Place your hips as far back as they will go in the chair while maintaining a comfortable sitting position. Check that the chair's back is firmly attached to the backrest.
4. Maintain a tight core by contracting the abs and lumbar region. Put some space between your ribs.

5. Always ensure that both palms are facing down and that your elbows are bent

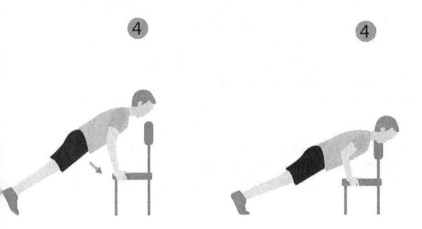

and parallel to your shoulders. Both hands should be positioned so that they are just outside of the breadth of the shoulder.

6. Don't bring your hands together as you stretch your arms fully in front of the body while doing this exercise; push the resistance band forward.

7. Bring yourself back to the starting position slowly.

Note: If a chair cannot be altered to accommodate the resistance band or insufficient tension, the band can be wrapped around another stable device such as a pole or beam.

Modified Push-Ups

Complicacy	Reps /Sets	Minimum Time
Advanced	8-12/2-3	5 minutes

Steps:

1. Stand with your body aligned to face the chair straight.

2. Put both hands on the chair's armrests for a more secure grip. While keeping both arms in a position where the elbows are slightly bent, move both feet backward a couple of feet until the body is in a position where it is diagonal to the chair. Check that your back is not arched and your buttocks are not raised too high. Heel shoulder should form a straight line. The body should be in this position. When seniors feel resistance or stress in their core, they are in the appropriate position. It is recommended that the elbows be brought close to the body's sides.
3. Bending the elbows slowly will bring the body closer to the chair.
4. Push yourself back to the beginning position as soon as your chin almost touches the chair or as close to the chair as you can.

Note that positioning the chair against a wall provides additional support. During this activity, if the chair is not put against a wall, you should take precautions to ensure it will not slide. Be careful when holding onto the chair because your sweaty palms could cause you to lose your grip.

Bicep

Two separate muscle heads make up the bicep in each of our bodies. We can pick things up and bring them closer to our bodies if we have strong biceps. Most of the movements we do with our arms involve our biceps, yet we do so for reasons distinct from those served by our shoulders.

Supine Bicep Curls (Seated)

Complicacy	Reps /Sets	Minimum Time
Easy	8-12/2-3	4 minutes

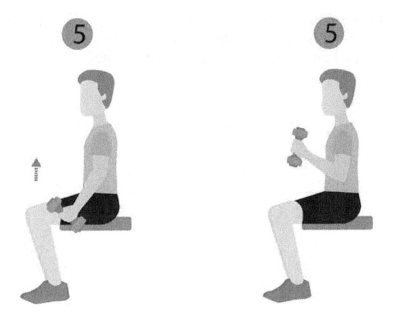

Steps:

1. Grab a set of dumbbells or a resistance band.
2. If you use a resistance band, slide it beneath the seat or sit on it until it is the same length on both sides of your body.
3. Take a comfortable seat in the chair, moving your hips as far back as they go. Check that the back is securely fastened to the chair's backrest.
4. Maintain a tightness in the core, including the lumbar region and the abdominals. Put your chest out there.
5. Maintain both arms at your sides, let them hang naturally with your palms facing forward, and tuck your elbows close to your sides (at the sides of your body).
6. Proceed to move both forearms in a curling motion from the sides of the body to the front of the shoulders (the senior does not need to touch their hands to their shoulders for a full range of motion).
7. While maintaining tension, return both forearms to their initial position as you progressively lower them.

Triceps

Although the triceps do not play a significant role in lifting objects, seniors who are self-conscious about dangling under-arm skin (whether due to excess skin or fat) and who want to tighten this area will find that triceps exercises are very helpful.

Isolated Triceps Extensions

Complicacy	Reps /Sets	Minimum Time
Medium	8-12/2-3	7 minutes

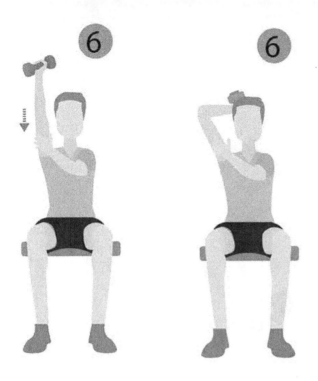

If you've been working on developing shoulder motion, you'll find that this exercise is much simpler to perform.

Steps:

1. Grab a dumbbell.
2. Place your hips as far back as they will go in the chair while maintaining a comfortable sitting position. Check that the chair's back is firmly attached to the backrest.
3. Maintain a tight core by contracting the abs and lumbar region. Put some space between your ribs.
4. Maintain a "V" form by keeping both elbows up and in front of the body while lowering one hand behind the head to create space. Make use of your other hand to provide support for the arm slightly below the elbow. Maintain the position of the assisting hand here (without applying too much pressure). It is proper form to have the palm holding a dumbbell facing upwards toward the body.
5. Raise one arm while holding a dumbbell over your head until it is fully extended.
6. Bring the forearm back to the beginning position in a controlled manner.
7. It should be repeated for both arms.

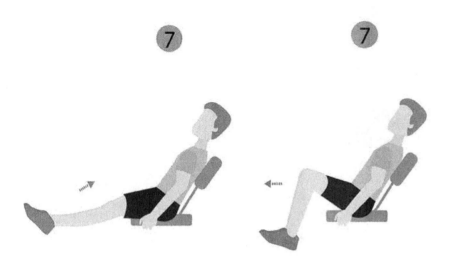

SECTION TWO

Core Exercises

The center of everything we accomplish throughout the day is the most important component. We engage our core muscles whenever we are upright, whether walking, stooping, standing, or even sitting. If we do not engage our core muscles to maintain appropriate posture, we run the risk of slouching our back, which can lead to muscle strain and other problems of a similar nature.

Knee-to-Chest

Complicacy	Reps /Sets	Minimum Time
Easy	8-12/2-3	4 minutes

Steps:

1. You should be able to sit at the edge of the chair without feeling as though you are going to topple over.

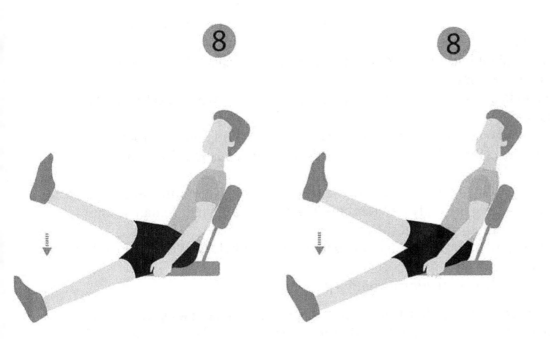

2. Maintain a straight back while contracting the core muscles (abs and lumbar). Put some space between your ribs.
3. Put both hands on the side of the chair, then grab the seat with both to maintain your balance.
4. Put both feet a good distance in front of the body, and then point the toes of both feet toward the ceiling. Both feet must be perpendicular to the hips.
5. While bending your knees, slowly bring both legs into a position where they are closer to the body. Bring both knees as near as they can to the center of your chest.
6. Move slowly through this motion, but this time perform it in the other direction, back into the starting position. One "rep" is equal to this amount.

Note that you may also perform this movement by isolating it one leg at a time. Before lifting, check that the leg that will not be supporting your weight is firmly placed on the ground.

Extended Leg Raises

Complicacy	Reps /Sets	Minimum Time
Medium	8-12/2-3	4 minutes

Steps:

1. You should be able to sit at the edge of the chair without feeling as though you are going to topple over.
2. Maintain a straight back while contracting the core muscles (abs and lumbar). Put some space between your ribs.
3. Put both hands on the side of the chair, then grab the seat with both to maintain your balance.
4. Put both feet a good distance in front of the body, and then point the toes of both feet toward the ceiling. Both of your feet have to be in a perpendicular position to your hips.
5. Raise one leg to the highest point possible (the ideal range of motion ends at the hips) while keeping the body's center still. The opposite leg will remain in the beginning position throughout the exercise.
6. Return the leg to the starting position by lowering it slowly, and then repeat the process with the other leg.
7. One "rep" is equivalent to kicking both legs.

Take note that you can also perform this movement by focusing on just one leg at a time. Before elevating the leg, double-check that the other leg is firmly placed on the ground.

Leg Kicks

Complicacy	Reps /Sets	Minimum Time
Advance	8-12/2-3	5 minutes

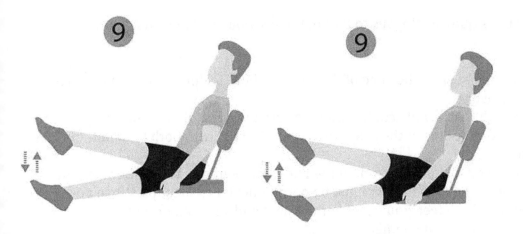

The motion of this exercise is quite analogous to that of the previously extended leg lifts.

Steps:

1. You should be able to sit at the edge of the chair without feeling as though you are going to topple over.
2. Maintain a straight back while contracting the core muscles (abs and lumbar).
3. Put both hands on the side of the chair, then grab the seat with both to maintain your balance.
4. Put both feet a good distance in front of the body and point the toes of both feet in the direction of the body. Both feet must be perpendicular to the hips. When you step forward with both feet, you should gradually bend your upper body backward to support the movement.
5. Raise one leg to the top of its range of motion to reach a position in which it is parallel to the hips. Do this without moving the core of the body.
6. After returning one leg to its starting position in a controlled manner, switch to the other leg. Imagine the individual swimming and kicking their legs in the water as they perform this movement. This is a helpful mental image to have.
7. One "rep" equals one kick performed on each leg.

Note: If you want to make this exercise more difficult for yourself, attempt to avoid touching your feet to the ground until the very end of the exercise. This action can also be broken down into parts using one leg at a time. Before lifting, double-check that the leg that will not be supporting your weight is firmly placed on the ground.

Modified Planks

Complicacy	Reps /Sets	Minimum Time
Advance	30/2-3 seconds	4 minutes

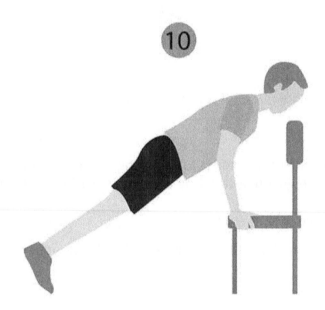

One of the most well-known and effective exercises for the abdominal core, planks can be performed by people of any age. Because of the workout, more tension is placed on the core, which causes the body to remain stable. Maintaining a healthy posture when seated is one of the many benefits that this action may attain through practice.

Steps:

1. Stand with your body aligned to face the chair straight.
2. Put both hands on the chair's armrests for a more secure grip. While keeping both arms in a position where the elbows are slightly bent, move both feet backward a couple of feet until the body is in a position where it is diagonal to the chair. Check to see that your back is not arched and your buttocks are not raised too high. Heel shoulder should form a straight line. The body should be in this position. When seniors feel resistance or stress in their core, they are in the appropriate position.

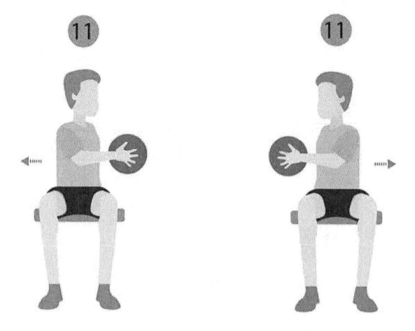

3. Hold this position for thirty seconds (or for as long as it is comfortable without causing pain), and then go into a standing or seated position to give yourself a little break.
4. **It should be done twice or three times.**

Note that positioning the chair against a wall provides additional support.

Tummy Twists

Complicacy	Reps /Sets	Minimum Time
Medium	8-10/2-3	5 minutes

This exercise targets the entire core and helps extend the spine simultaneously, making it a well-rounded core workout. This exercise should be performed for maximum strain in the abdominal region using a medicine ball or another item with a similar shape.

Steps:

1. Grab a medicine ball (or similar object).
2. Place yourself in the chair so that you are facing the edge of the seat. This will provide you with additional space. Maintain a tight core by contracting the abs and lumbar region. Put some space between your ribs. The elbows should be bent, and the hands should be placed in front of the body, so they are clutching the sides of the medicine ball.

3. Raise the ball a few centimeters above the ground and twist your upper body to the right while maintaining the ball's position in front of your torso.
4. Rotate to the middle of the body, then rotate to the left, and finally, back to the middle to complete the movement.
5. One "rep" corresponds to one complete rotation.

SECTION THREE

Leg Exercises

We make all of our migratory movements during the day using only our legs unless we are confined to a wheelchair or are undergoing some other condition. Utilizing our legs entails standing, walking, jogging, ascending stairs, and bending down to pick things up from the ground. As we become older, one of the important physical considerations we need to give attention to is maintaining our leg strength.

But activities such as jogging, running, and climbing stairs can tax the joints, particularly for older seniors who have knee injuries or have had knee surgery within the past few months. Therefore, employing activities that can be done in a chair can help maintain leg strength and endurance while protecting the joints.

Make sure you have the appropriate footwear before you begin the below workouts! You won't believe how important the right shoes can be when working out. Even if the person you care about does not engage in activities such as jogging, hiking, or lifting heavy weights, they will still want shoes that provide cushioning (for comfort) and assistance with stability. Suppose they are doing anything resembling a squat. In that case, wearing flat shoes can be of assistance in maintaining a straight back and aligned knees rather than collapsing (buckling) inward into the body's midline. This is an undesirable movement pattern that should be avoided.

Sit-to-Stands (aka Chair Squat)

Complicacy	Reps /Sets	Minimum Time
Easy	8-12/2-3	5 minutes

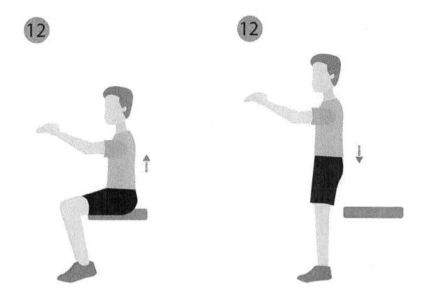

This exercise should start with the older adult using their body weight as the resistance. If they have the impression that it is too simple and their body enjoys the action, they can increase the difficulty by adding weight by carrying a medicine ball or another object of equivalent weight.

Steps:

1. Place yourself in a relaxed position toward the outer edge of the chair's seat.
2. Maintain a tight core by contracting the abs and lumbar region. Put some space between your ribs.
3. To maintain your balance, ensure that your toes are pointing forward or slightly outward to both sides, and keep both hands in front of your body in a comfortable posture.
4. Begin to slowly rise from the chair until you are standing completely. When transitioning from sitting to standing, ensure that your knees are not bowing inward; instead, they should be extending outward from the center of your body. When performing this exercise, the knees should not be used to propel the body into a standing position; rather, the hips should be used.
5. To return to the starting position, sit back down and double-check the positioning of your knees.

Note: If you want to tone your glutes (buttocks), you should squeeze them together when moving from sitting to standing. This will engage the glutes more and get you started on the path to muscle toning.

Modified Squats

Complicacy	Reps /Sets	Minimum Time
Medium	8-12/2-3	5 minutes

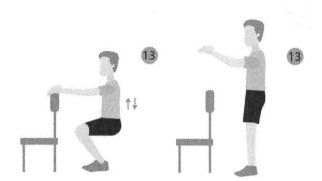

Squatting is considered one of the most beneficial workouts that a person of any age can practice, and this is true regardless of age. However, a normal squat is not something everyone can do, and there are situations when assistance is required.

Steps:

1. Place the chair in front of the body with the back of the chair towards the rear of the body. Take one step backward from where you are sitting on the chair.
2. Position the body, so it is centered directly in the middle of the chair. Put both hands in a prayer position in front of your body.
3. Place both feet precisely under the torso, hip-width apart, and in a vertical position.
4. Toes can be pointed forward or in a somewhat distant direction from the body's center.
5. While maintaining the position of the knees behind the toes (do not allow them to cross over the toes), bend both knees, release the hips, and lower the buttocks toward the ground. Keep a close eye on both knees to ensure they do not cave inward into the middle of the body; instead, drive them outward away from you.
6. After stopping in the squat position, you should immediately push your body up into a standing position.

Note: If the chair is swaying or wobbling, you can improve its stability by bracing its front end against a wall. In addition, if the back of the chair is tall, you can secure yourself by placing your hands on the very top of it.

Knee Extensions

Complicacy	Reps /Sets	Minimum Time
Easy	8-12/2-3	6 minutes

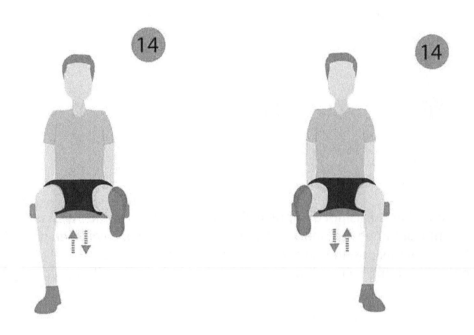

Steps:

1. Place your hips as far back as they will go in the chair while maintaining a comfortable sitting position. Check that the chair's back is firmly attached to the backrest.
2. Maintain a tight core by contracting the abs and lumbar region. Put some space between your ribs.
3. Put both hands on the side of the chair, then grab the seat with both to maintain your balance.
4. Always maintain a 90-degree angle between both of your legs and the chair.
5. Perform a full extension of one leg in front of the torso, raising it as far as possible. For stability, you should maintain the position of the other leg.
6. Bring one leg back to the starting position as slowly as possible.

It will count as one set if you repeat that for both legs.

Heel Slides

Complicacy	Reps /Sets	Minimum Time
Easy	8-12/2-3	6 minutes

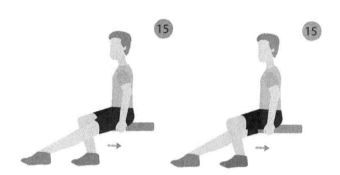

Due to the pressure exerted on the joints, it is possible that this is not an appropriate workout for a senior who is currently dealing with significant knee discomfort. If an older person does have knee pain, they should apply as little pressure as possible to avoid irritating the joint. Take a towel or a blanket and position it so that it is lying on the floor in front of the chair. This will prevent any harm to the floor.

Steps:

1. Place yourself in a relaxed position toward the outer edge of the chair's seat.
2. Maintain a tight core by contracting the abs and lumbar region. Put some space between your ribs.
3. Put both hands on the side of the chair, then grab the seat with both to maintain your balance.
4. Extend one leg in front of the torso as far as you can and point the toes forward. The foot of the extended leg should be angled diagonally to the hips. If you are using a blanket or another object, position it so that the foot is on top. The other leg should be naturally bent, close to the body, with the foot planted on the floor.
5. Keep the foot of the leg extended in a flat position, apply pressure to the floor, and gradually bring the extended foot closer to the body until it reaches the flexed position of the other leg.
6. Maintaining the pressure, bring the leg back to the beginning position as you stretch it.
7. A single repetition is accomplished by completing the whole movement, which consists of pulling and pushing the foot back to the beginning.

Seated Calf Raises

Complicacy	Reps /Sets	Minimum Time
Easy	20-30/3	6 minutes

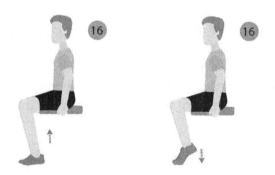

If a senior feels tense in their calves and it isn't very easy to squat, calf raises might help stretch those tense muscles or joints around the lower part of the leg.

Steps:

1. Sit comfortably in the chair with the hips as far back as possible. Ensure that the back is firm to the backrest of the chair.
2. Keep the core (abs and lumbar) tight. Stick the chest out.
3. Place both hands at the sides of the chair and grip the seat to keep it stable.
4. Keep both legs at a 90-degree angle with the chair. Both feet should be flat on the floor.
5. Slowly extend the heels of your feet upward, pushing the toes on the ground and lifting the heels in the air.
6. Place both feet back to the starting position.
7. Repeat this movement for 20 or more reps to create a "burning" feeling in the calves.

Note: If this movement feels too easy with just bodyweight, place a medicine ball or another weight of equal value towards the edge of the lap (almost to the knees). Or, put an external object underneath both feet (about 3-4 inches off the ground) for a full range of motion.

SECTION FOUR

Stretching Exercises

The practice of stretching is of utmost significance. Because there are so many benefits to keeping the body flexible and relaxed, especially after performing the exercises described above, not a single personal trainer or physical therapist will ever say that stretching is a bad idea when it comes to exercise. Stretching helps keep the body flexible and relaxed, which helps the body perform better. There are many different ways to stretch, and all of them are healthy in their own right.

A wide variety of flexibility training may be carried out when the individual is standing or lying on the ground. Certain stretches for the upper back can most certainly assist with some of the exercises described earlier in this guide.

On the other hand, if you can't perform the stretches on the floor, don't worry; we have some chair stretches ready and waiting for you. Altering certain other stretches so that you do them while seated on a chair provides an additional degree of stability.

How Frequently Should an Older Person Stretch?

If you are above the age of 50, you should stretch anywhere from two to five times each week, depending on the tension and mobility you require.

Compared to the number of times stretching is done throughout the day, the amount of time spent stretching does not necessarily have any bearing on its benefits. Put aside around ten to fifteen minutes a day to complete the stretches on your own. When they stretch, they should do it with patience and focus on taking deep breaths to calm both their body and mind.

When to Stretch

The question of when people should do their stretching during the day has been the subject of much discussion. There isn't a consensus amongst fitness experts and medical specialists regarding the optimal time of day for an individual to stretch and when they should.

Neck Turns

Complicacy	Reps /Sets	Minimum Time
Easy	20-30/3-5	5 minutes

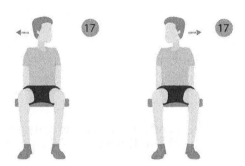

A stiff neck is quite uncomfortable. If a senior isn't getting sufficient sleep due to pain in their neck or can't swivel their head easily, extending it might ease the discomfort.

Steps:

1. Sit comfortably in the chair with the hips as far back as possible. Ensure that the back is solid to the backrest of the chair. Secure the core by maintaining the back upright and the spine straight. Keep both feet flat on the floor.
2. Keeping in this position, swivel the head to either the left or right until experiencing a slight stretch. Keep in this position for 20-30 seconds.
3. After the time passes, rotate in the opposite direction.
4. Repeat in both directions 3-5 times or as comfortable.

Seated Backbend

Complicacy	Reps /Sets	Minimum Time
Easy	10-20/3-5	4 minutes

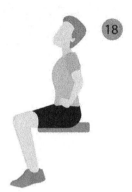

This stretch is ideal for seniors experiencing pain or tightness in their lower back, neck, or chest. It targets all three areas.

Steps:

1. Place yourself in a relaxed position on the chair's edge. Protect the vital organs by maintaining a vertical back and a straight spine. Maintain a flat footing on both feet on the floor. Maintain this secure position with the hips and the rest of the lower body.
2. Put both hands on your hips while you do so.
3. After slowly arching the back inward while pulling the stomach outward, leaning backward using only the upper body will produce the desired effect.
4. The back should be extended to the point where a comfortable stretch is reached in this position.
5. Hold this position for ten to twenty seconds, then relax and return to the starting position.
6. Repeat the pattern three to five times or until it seems natural.

Seated Overhead Stretch

Complicacy	Reps /Sets	Minimum Time
Easy	10-20/3-5	4 minutes

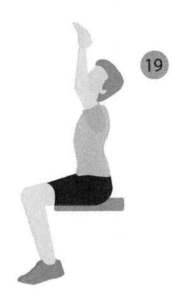

Steps:

1. Place yourself in a relaxed position on the chair's edge. Protect the vital organs by maintaining a vertical back and a straight spine. Maintain a flat footing on both feet on the floor. Maintain this secure position with the hips and the rest of the lower body.
2. Put both hands on your hips while you do so.
3. Raise both hands slowly over the head from the hips, then interlock both hands' fingers at the movement's peak.
4. Make a small inward arch in the back while also pulling the stomach outward to create a stretch in the abdominal region.
5. This position should be held for 10–20 seconds before returning to the starting position.
6. Perform the exercise three to five times or until you feel comfortable stopping.

Seated Side Stretch

Complicacy	Reps /Sets	Minimum Time
Medium	10-20/3-5	8 minutes

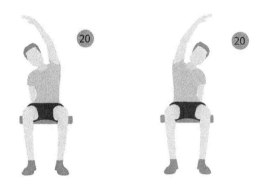

Steps:

1. Place yourself in a relaxed position on the chair's edge. Protect the vital organs by maintaining a vertical back and a straight spine. Maintain a flat footing on both feet on the floor. Maintain this secure position with the hips and the rest of the lower body.
2. Grab the right side of the seat with your right hand to help you stabilize yourself.
3. Extend the left hand over the head in a shape comparable to that of a spoon or a "C" that has been elongated.
4. At the same time, rotate your upper torso to the right in a controlled manner without bending your abdominal muscles (keep it tight).
5. Keep the position for ten to twenty seconds, and then switch sides.
6. Repeat three to five times on each side or as many times as is comfortable.

Seated Hip Stretch

Complicacy	Reps /Sets	Minimum Time
Medium	10-20/3-5	8 minutes

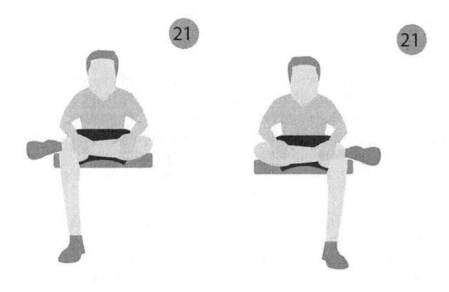

The hips play a significant role in the actions that we do daily. If a senior is slouching, has difficulty moving their legs at the hips, feels like they are waddling when they walk or has a pattern of pain in the general area of their hips, they may find that this stretch is beneficial.

Steps:

1. Please make yourself at home in the chair. Protect the vital organs by maintaining a vertical back and a straight spine. Maintain a flat footing on both feet on the floor.
2. You should now have a triangle formed between your legs by crossing one leg over the other. Check to see that the ankle of the leg that is crossed is in front of the other leg.
3. Move the upper body forward in a slow, controlled motion while maintaining a straight spine and a firm core. Stop the exercise when you feel resistance in your glutes or your hips.
4. Maintain this position for ten to twenty seconds, and then switch sides.
5. Repeat three to five times or as often as comfortably per leg.

Conclusion

Because overexerting oneself in any of the actions mentioned above might result in injury or even worse, persons over 50 should avoid doing so at all costs. They shouldn't put any further pressure on their body if it's rejecting any of the moves that are being suggested. When we push our bodies physically, they communicate with us, letting us know when something is a good idea and when it is a bad idea. Every part of our body is linked together by a chain of muscles, and just like any other chain, if one of these links becomes weak, the others will not function in the same way.

If an elderly person or their caregiver is working toward establishing a better habit, nutrition should also be an aspect that corresponds with the workouts being performed. Seniors need to incorporate nutritious meals and snacks into their daily routines because these foods can even help improve energy levels when seniors are feeling fatigued. If a senior wants to get the most out of these chair exercises, they need to pay attention to what their body is telling them. When executing any of the activities on the list, it is perfectly acceptable to seek assistance or proceed more slowly than is customary.